Time To Trim Down

Transform Your Body In No Time

Gloria R. Brewer

Acknowledgements

Writing "Time to Trim Down" has been a journey of self-discovery, growth, and transformation, and I am deeply grateful to all those who have supported and inspired me along the way.

First and foremost, I would like to express my heartfelt gratitude to the pioneers and experts in the field of weight loss and wellness whose work has informed and inspired my own. Thank you to Dr.Jason Fung, whose groundbreaking research and insights have shed light on the complex relationship between nutrition,

metabolism, and weight management. Your contributions to the field have been invaluable, and I am honored to have benefited from your wisdom and expertise.

I would also like to extend my gratitude to Dr.Michael Mosley, whose innovative approaches to emotional eating and behavior change have been a source of inspiration and motivation for me. Your compassionate approach to wellness has touched the lives of countless individuals, myself included, and I am grateful for the guidance and support you have provided.

To my family, whose unwavering love and support have been my rock throughout this journey, I am eternally grateful.

Thank you for standing by me, cheering me on, and believing in me even when I doubted myself. Your encouragement have meant the world to me, and I am endlessly thankful for the sacrifices you have made to help me pursue my dreams. To my friends and colleagues, thank you for your words of the encouragement, your words of wisdom, and your unwavering belief in my abilities. Your support has been a constant source of strength and inspiration, and I am grateful for the laughter, the camaraderie, and the shared moments of joy and celebration.

Finally, to the readers of "Time to Trim Down," thank you for embarking on this journey with me. Whether you are just beginning your own transformation or are well on your way, I hope that this book serves as a source of inspiration, guidance, and encouragement as you work towards your health and wellness goals. Remember, you are capable of achieving greatness, and with dedication, perseverance, and a little help from those who believe in you, anything is possible.

With deepest gratitude,

Gloria R. Brewer

About the Author

Gloria R. Brewer is not just a chef, but a passionate advocate for healthy eating and sustainable weight loss. With a background in culinary arts and a deep-seated commitment to wellness,Gloria R. Brewer brings a unique perspective to the table—one that blends culinary expertise with a deep understanding of nutrition and wellness.

From a young age,Gloria R. Brewer discovered her love for cooking and the transformative power of food. Inspired by the vibrant flavors and rich traditions of her cultural heritage, she embarked on a journey to explore the world of culinary arts, honing her skills in kitchens both near and far.

But it wasn't until Gloria R. Brewer faced her own struggles with weight and health that her passion for cooking took on a new dimension. Determined to reclaim her vitality and well-being, she immersed herself in the study of nutrition, seeking out the latest research and insights on weight loss and healthy eating.

Armed with this knowledge,Gloria R. Brewer began to experiment in the kitchen, creating delicious, nutritious meals that nourished her body and soul. Through trial and error, she discovered the power of whole, unprocessed foods to support weight loss, boost energy levels, and improve overall health.

Now, as a chef and wellness advocate,Gloria R. Brewer is on a mission to share her passion for healthy eating with the world. Through her books, cooking classes, and online platforms, she empowers others to take control of their health and transform their lives, one delicious meal at a time.

With a focus on fresh, seasonal ingredients and innovative cooking techniques,Gloria R. Brewer inspires readers to get creative in the kitchen and discover the joy of cooking for health and happiness. Whether you're a seasoned chef or a novice cook,Gloria R. Brewer's recipes and insights are sure to inspire and delight, guiding you on your own journey to vibrant health and wellness.

Join Gloria R. Brewer on this culinary adventure and discover the transformative power of food to nourish your body, uplift your spirit, and create a life filled with vitality and joy.

CONTENT

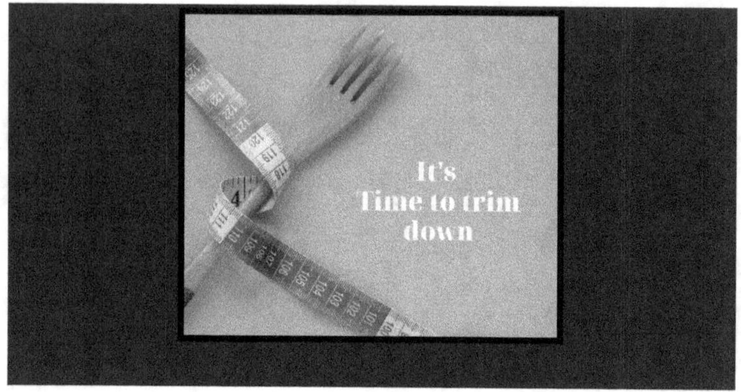

INTRODUCTION

In the bustling heart of the city,where the streets hummed with the rhythm of life, there stood a figure. She was like so many others, navigating the urban landscape with purpose and determination. Yet, beneath the facade of confidence, there lurked a shadow—a weight that she carried with her, both literal and metaphorical.

Her name was Sonia, and like so many of us, she had found herself trapped in a cycle of frustration and despair. For years, she had struggled with her weight, battling against the relentless tide of diets, exercise plans, and empty promises. Each day seemed to blur into the next, as she fought against her own body, desperate to reclaim the vitality and confidence she knew she deserved.

But despite her best efforts, the numbers on the scale refused to budge, and Sonia found herself sinking deeper into despair. She watched as friends and colleagues effortlessly shed pounds, their bodies transforming before her eyes, while she remained stuck in the same old rut.

It was in the depths of this despair that Sonia stumbled upon a glimmer of hope—a book with a title that seemed to speak directly to her soul: "Time to Trim Down." Intrigued, she flipped through the pages, devouring each word with a hunger she hadn't felt in years. Here, finally, was a roadmap to a brighter future—a guide that promised to unlock the secrets of sustainable weight loss and lasting transformation.

As Sonia delved deeper into the pages of "Time to Trim Down," she found herself captivated by the stories of others who had walked the same path. From overcoming emotional eating to demystifying metabolism, each chapter offered a new revelation, a fresh perspective on the journey she had embarked upon.

But it was not just the practical advice that drew Sonia in—it was the underlying message of empowerment and self-love that resonated most deeply. Here was a book that didn't just promise to help her shed pounds—it promised to help her reclaim her life, to rediscover the joy and vitality that had been lost to her for so long. With renewed determination, Sonia set out to put the principles of "Time to Trim Down" into practice. Armed with knowledge and inspiration, she began to make small changes in her daily life, swapping out processed foods for whole, nutrient-dense options, and finding joy in movement and exercise once again.

And as the days turned into weeks and the weeks into months, Sonia watched in amazement as the numbers on the scale began to shift. But more than that, she felt a transformation taking place within herself—a newfound sense of confidence, resilience, and self-love that radiated from every pore.

Now, as Sonia stands on the threshold of a new chapter in her life, she knows that the journey is far from over. But armed with the lessons and insights she has gained from "Time to Trim Down," she faces the future with courage and optimism, knowing that she has the power to create the life she's always dreamed of.

Dear reader, if you find yourself standing where Sonia once stood—trapped in a cycle of frustration and despair—I invite you to join us on this journey of transformation. Let "Time to Trim Down" be your guide, your companion, and your inspiration as you reclaim your health, your happiness, and your life. The road ahead may be long and challenging, but with courage, determination, and a little help from this book, anything is possible.

CHAPTER 1:
UNDERSTANDING YOUR RELATIONSHIP WITH FOOD

Recognizing Patterns and Triggers

Recognizing patterns and triggers is a crucial aspect of understanding our relationship with food and ultimately achieving successful weight management. Let's delve into this topic extensively:

Understanding Patterns:

Patterns refer to recurring behaviors, thoughts, or actions that occur consistently over time. When it comes to our eating habits, patterns can manifest in various ways. These could include:

- **Eating Schedule:** Pay attention to when you typically eat throughout the day. Are there specific times when you tend to feel hungry or snack more frequently?

- **Food Choices:** Notice the types of foods you commonly crave or consume. Are there certain food groups or specific foods that you gravitate towards during stressful times or particular emotions?

- **Environmental Triggers:** Consider the environments or situations that often prompt you to eat. This could be at social gatherings, while watching TV, or when passing by certain food outlets.
- **Emotional Triggers:** Explore the connection between your emotions and eating habits. Do you find yourself turning to food for comfort, stress relief, or as a price?

Identifying Triggers:

Triggers are stimuli or cues that prompt certain behaviors or reactions.

In the context of eating, triggers can be categorized into various types:

- **Emotional Triggers:** These are emotions or mood states that lead to eating. Examples include stress, boredom, sadness, loneliness, anxiety, or even happiness.
- **Environmental Triggers:** These are external factors in your surroundings that stimulate the desire to eat. They can include sights, smells, sounds, or social situations that evoke cravings or appetitive responses.
- **Social Triggers:** Interactions with others, social norms, or peer pressure can influence eating behaviors. For example, you might find yourself eating more in social settings to fit in or as a form of bonding with others.
- **Habitual Triggers:** Certain routines or habits can trigger eating behaviors almost automatically, without conscious awareness. These could include habits like snacking while watching TV or grabbing a sugary treat after dinner.

Strategies for Recognition and Management:

- **Self-Awareness:** Cultivate mindfulness and self-awareness around your eating habits. Keep a food diary to track when, what, and why you eat. This can help identify patterns and triggers.

- **Emotional Regulation:** Develop alternative coping mechanisms for managing emotions without turning to food. Practice stress-relief techniques such as deep breathing, meditation, or engaging in hobbies or activities you enjoy.

- **Modify Your Environment:** Make changes to your physical surroundings to minimize exposure to food triggers. For example, keep unhealthy snacks out of sight, stock your kitchen with nutritious options, and create a supportive environment for your wellness goals.

- **Seek Support:** Share your goals and challenges with supportive friends, family members, or a healthcare professional. They can provide encouragement, accountability, and practical strategies for dealing with triggers.

By recognizing patterns and triggers related to your eating habits, you gain greater insight and control over your behaviors. With this awareness, you can develop healthier coping mechanisms, make more mindful food choices, and ultimately achieve your weight management goals

Understanding patterns and triggers in our eating habits is akin to deciphering the intricate puzzle of our relationship with food. It involves peeling back the layers of our behavior to reveal the underlying motivations and influences that drive our dietary choices. By delving into the depths of our eating patterns, we uncover valuable insights into our habits, preferences, and vulnerabilities.

Our eating patterns are like the threads woven into the fabric of our daily lives, guiding us through the rhythms of breakfast, lunch, and dinner. They are the rituals we enact, the routines we follow, and the habits we form over time. Whether it's reaching for a mid-afternoon snack out of habit or indulging in dessert after dinner as a reward, these patterns shape our eating behaviors in profound ways.

Triggers, on the other hand, are the catalysts that ignite our desire to eat. They can be external stimuli that beckon us from the confines of our environment or internal cues that arise from within. Perhaps it's the aroma of freshly baked bread wafting from a nearby bakery, the sight of a mouth-watering dessert on a restaurant menu, or the subtle pang of loneliness that creeps in during moments of solitude. These triggers have the power to pull us towards food, often without us even realizing it.

Recognizing these patterns and triggers requires a keen sense of self-awareness and soul-searching. It's about tuning into the subtle nuances of our thoughts, emotions, and behaviors, and making connections between them. By becoming attuned to the patterns that govern our eating habits and the triggers that set them in motion, we empower ourselves to make more conscious choices about what, when, and why we eat.

Moreover, understanding patterns and triggers is not merely about identifying them; it's also about learning how to navigate them effectively. It's about developing strategies to manage cravings, cope with stress, and resist temptation in the face of triggers. Whether it's practicing mindfulness techniques to cultivate greater awareness in the present moment or finding alternative outlets for emotional expression, there are myriad ways we can harness our newfound understanding to support our health and well-being.

Ultimately, recognizing patterns and triggers in our eating habits is a journey of self-discovery and transformation. It's about peeling back the layers of habit and impulse to reveal the true drivers of our behavior. By shining a light on these hidden forces, we gain the power to rewrite our stories, forge new pathways, and reclaim control over our relationship with food. In doing so, we pave the way for a healthier, happier, and more fulfilling life.

Overcoming Emotional Eating

Overcoming emotional eating is a multifaceted journey that involves understanding the complex interplay between our emotions and our relationship with food. At its core, emotional eating is the act of using food as a coping mechanism to deal with difficult emotions, such as stress, anxiety, sadness, boredom, or even happiness. Rather than eating in response to physical hunger, emotional eating is driven by psychological factors and often leads to overeating or consuming unhealthy foods.

One of the first steps in overcoming emotional eating is recognizing and acknowledging the patterns and triggers that contribute to this behavior. This requires developing a heightened awareness of our emotions and the role they play in our eating habits. By paying attention to the thoughts, feelings, and situations that precede episodes of emotional eating, we can begin to unravel the underlying reasons behind our behavior.

Once we've identified the triggers for emotional eating, the next step is to develop alternative coping mechanisms for managing our emotions without turning to food. This might involve practicing mindfulness techniques, such as deep breathing, meditation, or progressive muscle relaxation, to help us become more present and grounded in the moment. By cultivating greater awareness of our internal experiences, we can learn to observe our emotions without automatically resorting to food as a form of comfort or distraction.

Another effective strategy for overcoming emotional eating is to build a toolbox of healthy coping mechanisms that we can turn to in times of distress. This might include engaging in physical activity, such as going for a walk, practicing yoga, or dancing to our favorite music, as a way to release pent-up tension and stress. Similarly, engaging in creative activities, such as writing, painting, or gardening, can provide a constructive outlet for processing emotions and channeling our energy in positive ways.

As well, developing a strong support network can be instrumental in overcoming emotional eating. Whether it's confiding in a trusted friend, family member, or therapist, having someone to turn to for encouragement, guidance, and accountability can make a world of difference. Additionally, joining a support group or seeking professional help from a therapist who specializes in disordered eating can provide valuable resources and strategies for overcoming emotional eating.

It's important to recognize that overcoming emotional eating is not a linear process and may involve setbacks along the way. However, by approaching the journey with patience, compassion, and persistence, we can gradually develop healthier habits and patterns around food. By learning to nourish our bodies with self-care, compassion, and nutritious foods, rather than using food as a crutch to soothe our emotions, we can cultivate a more balanced and fulfilling relationship with food and ultimately reclaim control over our health and well-being.

Emotional eating is a complex phenomenon deeply rooted in the intricate dance between our mind and body. It's a behavior that often arises from a desire to find solace, comfort, or distraction in food during times of emotional upheaval. Whether it's stress from work, relationship troubles, or simply feeling overwhelmed by life's challenges, food can become a source of refuge—a temporary reprieve from the storm of our emotions.

However, while emotional eating may provide momentary relief, it often comes at a cost. Over time, relying on food as a coping mechanism can lead to a host of negative consequences, including weight gain, poor nutrition, and feelings of guilt or shame. What begins as a fleeting escape from emotional discomfort can spiral into a cycle of overeating, followed by remorse and self-recrimination.

To break free from the grip of emotional eating, it's essential to cultivate a deeper understanding of our emotional landscape. This involves learning to recognize and accept our feelings, even the uncomfortable ones, without judgment or suppression. By tuning into the subtle signals of our emotions—whether it's the tightness in our chest, the knot in our stomach, or the heaviness in our heart—we can begin to unravel the tangled web of thoughts and feelings that drive our urge to eat.

Moreover, overcoming emotional eating requires us to develop healthier ways of coping with our emotions. Rather than seeking solace in food, we can explore alternative strategies for self-soothing and emotional regulation. This might involve turning to activities that bring us joy, fulfillment, and a sense of connection, such as spending time with loved ones, pursuing hobbies, or practicing mindfulness and meditation.

It's important to cultivate a nourishing relationship with food—one that is based on self-care, balance, and mindfulness. This means tuning into our body's hunger and fullness cues, eating mindfully, and choosing foods that nourish and energize us. By honoring our body's needs and respecting its signals, we can begin to break free from the cycle of emotional eating and establish a more harmonious relationship with food.

CHAPTER 2:The Science of Weight Loss

Demystifying Metabolism

Demystifying metabolism is like shining a light into the dark corners of our body's inner workings, unraveling the mysterious processes that govern how we use energy and fuel our daily activities. Metabolism is often misunderstood, shrouded in myths and misconceptions, but at its core, it's a complex network of biochemical reactions that keep our bodies running smoothly.

At its simplest level, metabolism refers to the sum total of all the chemical processes that occur within our bodies to maintain life. This includes processes such as converting food into energy, building and repairing tissues, and eliminating waste products. Metabolism is a dynamic and highly regulated process that adapts to our changing needs, whether we're sprinting up a flight of stairs or lounging on the couch.

One of the biggest misconceptions about metabolism is that it's solely responsible for weight gain or loss. While metabolism does play a role in determining how many calories we burn at rest (known as basal metabolic rate), it's just one piece of the puzzle. Other factors, such as diet, physical activity, genetics, and hormonal balance, also influence our body composition and weight management.

Another common myth is that some people have a "fast" metabolism while others have a "slow" metabolism. While it's true that individual differences in metabolism exist, they're often exaggerated or misunderstood. Factors such as age, sex, muscle mass, and thyroid function can influence metabolic rate, but these differences are usually modest and can be offset through lifestyle modifications.

Understanding metabolism also involves dispelling myths about certain foods or dietary patterns that purportedly "boost" or "slow down" metabolism. While certain foods, such as spicy foods or caffeine, may temporarily increase metabolic rate, the effect is usually minimal and short-lived. Instead of fixating on specific foods or gimmicks, focusing on overall dietary patterns, such as eating a balanced diet rich in whole foods, is key to supporting metabolic health.

Besides, metabolism is not a static process—it's adaptable and responsive to our lifestyle habits. Regular physical activity, particularly strength training and high-intensity interval training, can increase muscle mass and boost metabolic rate over time. Similarly, getting an adequate amount of sleep, managing stress levels, and staying hydrated are all important factors for maintaining a healthy metabolism.

In essence, demystifying metabolism is about separating fact from fiction and empowering individuals to take control of their health and wellness. By understanding the fundamental principles of metabolism and how it interacts with our lifestyle choices, we can make informed decisions that support our overall well-being. Rather than viewing metabolism as a mysterious force beyond our control, we can embrace it as a dynamic and adaptable process that responds to the choices we make each day

Demystifying metabolism is like uncovering the hidden mechanisms that govern our body's energy expenditure and utilization. It's a journey of discovery, exploring the intricate biochemical pathways that transform food into fuel and power our every movement and thought.

One of the keys to understanding metabolism lies in grasping its multifaceted nature. Metabolism isn't a singular process but rather a complex web of interconnected reactions that occur within our cells and tissues. From breaking down carbohydrates, fats, and proteins to producing energy-rich molecules like adenosine triphosphate (ATP), metabolism is a finely tuned orchestra of biochemical activity.

Again, metabolism isn't confined to a specific organ or system but is distributed throughout the body. Organs such as the liver, muscles, and adipose tissue all play integral roles in metabolism, each contributing unique functions to the overall process. For example, the liver acts as a metabolic powerhouse, regulating blood sugar levels, synthesizing essential molecules, and detoxifying harmful substances.

Another aspect of metabolism that warrants exploration is its regulation and control. Metabolic pathways are tightly regulated by a complex network of hormones, enzymes, and signaling molecules that ensure balance and homeostasis within the body. For instance, hormones such as insulin and glucagon help regulate blood sugar levels by signaling cells to take up or release glucose as needed.

Furthermore, metabolism is highly adaptable and responsive to changes in our environment and lifestyle. For example, during periods of fasting or calorie restriction, metabolism slows down to conserve energy and preserve vital functions. Conversely, after a meal or during periods of physical activity, metabolism revs up to meet increased energy demands.

Understanding metabolism also involves debunking common myths and misconceptions that pervade popular culture. For instance, the idea of a "metabolic rate" that remains constant throughout life is a fallacy. Metabolic rate can vary widely from person to person and can fluctuate in response to factors such as age, sex, body composition, and activity level

Again, while genetics can influence metabolic tendencies to some extent, they're not the sole determinant of metabolic health. Lifestyle factors such as diet, exercise, sleep, and stress management play equally—if not more—significant roles in shaping metabolic function and overall health.

In essence, demystifying metabolism is about embracing curiosity and inquiry, delving into the intricate workings of our body's energy metabolism with a sense of wonder and fascination. By peeling back the layers of complexity and uncovering the underlying principles that govern metabolism, we empower ourselves to make informed choices that support our health, vitality, and well-being….

Establishing Realistic Goals

Establishing realistic goals is the cornerstone of any successful endeavor, whether it's embarking on a weight loss journey, pursuing a new career path, or striving to achieve personal growth. Realistic goals serve as guideposts, providing direction, motivation, and a sense of purpose as we navigate the ups and downs of life's journey.

At the heart of setting realistic goals lies the importance of self-awareness and introspection. It's about taking the time to reflect on our values, priorities, strengths, and limitations, and aligning our goals with our unique circumstances and aspirations. By acknowledging our starting point and understanding where we want to go, we can begin to chart a course that is both challenging and attainable.

Realistic goals are grounded in pragmatism and feasibility. They are achievable within a reasonable timeframe and are backed by a clear plan of action. Rather than setting lofty, unattainable goals that set us up for disappointment and frustration, realistic goals are within reach, yet still require effort, commitment, and perseverance to accomplish.

Moreover, realistic goals are specific and measurable, allowing us to track our progress and celebrate milestones along the way. Instead of vague aspirations like "lose weight" or "get in shape," realistic goals are concrete and tangible, such as "lose 10 pounds in three months" or "complete a 5K race in under 30 minutes." By breaking down larger goals into smaller, actionable steps, we make progress more manageable and attainable.

In addition, realistic goals are flexible and adaptable to changing circumstances. Life is unpredictable, and setbacks and obstacles are inevitable along the way. Rather than viewing setbacks as failures, realistic goals allow us to adjust our course, learn from our experiences, and continue moving forward with resilience and determination.

Again, establishing realistic goals involves cultivating a growth mindset—one that embraces challenges, learns from feedback, and persists in the face of adversity. Instead of viewing setbacks as insurmountable barriers, a growth mindset sees them as opportunities for learning and growth. By reframing setbacks as valuable lessons and opportunities for improvement, we can stay motivated and focused on our long-term goals.

Establishing realistic goals is not just about creating a checklist of tasks to accomplish; it's about embarking on a journey of self-discovery and growth. It's a process that requires introspection, reflection, and a willingness to challenge ourselves to reach new heights.

At its core, setting realistic goals involves striking a delicate balance between ambition and practicality. It's about dreaming big while also being mindful of our current circumstances and limitations. By setting goals that are both inspiring and attainable, we set ourselves up for success and avoid the pitfalls of overcommitment and burnout.

Again, establishing realistic goals requires us to consider the broader context of our lives. We must take into account factors such as our time commitments, financial resources, and personal obligations when crafting our goals. By being mindful of these constraints, we can ensure that our goals are not only achievable but also sustainable in the long run.

Realistic goals are also deeply rooted in self-awareness and self-compassion. It's important to be honest with ourselves about our strengths, weaknesses, and areas for improvement. By acknowledging our limitations without judgment, we can set goals that stretch us outside of our comfort zones while still being within the realm of possibility.

Furthermore, establishing realistic goals involves breaking down larger objectives into smaller, manageable steps. Rather than overwhelming ourselves with the enormity of our ambitions, we can focus on taking consistent, incremental actions that move us closer to our ultimate destination. By celebrating small victories along the way, we stay motivated and inspired to continue making progress.

In addition, realistic goals require us to cultivate resilience and adaptability. Setbacks and obstacles are inevitable on any journey, but it's how we respond to them that ultimately determines our success. By embracing failure as a natural part of the learning process and being willing to adjust our course when necessary, we demonstrate the resilience needed to overcome challenges and keep moving forward.

CHAPTER 3:Revolutionizing Your Diet

Navigating Nutrition Labels

Navigating nutrition labels is like decoding a secret language—a labyrinth of numbers, percentages, and unfamiliar terms that can leave even the most health-conscious consumers feeling bewildered. Yet, understanding how to read and interpret these labels is crucial for making informed choices about the foods we eat and supporting our overall health and well-being.

At its core, a nutrition label is a snapshot of the nutritional content of a food product. It provides valuable information about the serving size, calorie content, macronutrient composition, and key vitamins and minerals present in the food. By carefully examining these details, we can gain insights into the nutritional value of a product and make comparisons between different options.

One of the first things to look for when navigating a nutrition label is the serving size. This tells us the amount of food the nutrition information is based on and allows us to accurately assess the calorie and nutrient content of a single serving. It's important to note that the serving size listed on the label may not always correspond to the portion size we actually consume, so it's essential to adjust the information accordingly.

Next, it's helpful to examine the calorie content of the food. Calories provide a measure of the energy a food provides, and understanding how many calories are in a serving can help us manage our weight and make mindful choices about portion sizes. Additionally, the label may provide information about the breakdown of calories from carbohydrates, fats, and proteins, which can be useful for individuals following specific dietary patterns or health goals.

In addition to calories, nutrition labels typically include information about macronutrients such as carbohydrates, fats, and proteins. These macronutrients play essential roles in supporting various bodily functions and maintaining overall health. By paying attention to the amounts of carbohydrates, fats, and proteins in a food product, we can make choices that align with our nutritional needs and preferences.

Furthermore, nutrition labels often provide information about specific nutrients of concern, such as sodium, sugar, and dietary fiber. Monitoring our intake of these nutrients can help us make healthier choices and reduce our risk of chronic diseases such as heart disease, diabetes, and obesity. For example, choosing foods that are lower in sodium and added sugars and higher in fiber can contribute to better overall health.

Another aspect of navigating nutrition labels involves understanding the ingredient list. Ingredients are listed in descending order by weight, with the primary ingredient listed first. This can give us valuable insights into the composition of a food product and help us identify any potential allergens or additives that we may wish to avoid.

Also, it's important to be mindful of marketing claims and buzzwords that may appear on food packaging. Phrases such as "all-natural," "organic," or "low-fat" can be misleading and may not always reflect the true nutritional quality of a product. Instead, it's essential to rely on the information provided on the nutrition label to make informed decisions about the foods we consume.

Navigating nutrition labels is akin to unraveling the mysteries of the food we consume—a journey of discovery that empowers us to make informed choices about our diet and lifestyle. In today's world, where countless food products line the shelves of grocery stores, understanding how to decipher these labels is more important than ever.

One aspect of navigating nutrition labels that is often overlooked is the importance of context. While the label provides valuable information about the nutritional content of a food product, it's essential to consider how that information fits into our overall dietary pattern. For example, a food product that is high in fat or sugar may still have a place in a balanced diet if consumed in moderation and as part of a diverse array of foods.

Likewise, it's important to recognize that nutrition labels only tell part of the story when it comes to the healthfulness of a food product. While they provide information about the quantity of nutrients present, they may not always reflect the quality of those nutrients or the presence of other beneficial compounds such as antioxidants, phytochemicals, and fiber. Therefore, it's important to consider the broader nutritional profile of a food and how it fits into our overall dietary goals and preferences.

Also, navigating nutrition labels requires us to be critical consumers and question the information presented to us. While nutrition labels are regulated by government agencies and must adhere to certain standards, they can still be misleading or incomplete. For example, a food product labeled as "low-fat" may still be high in sugar or sodium, and vice versa. By being discerning and looking beyond the marketing hype, we can make more informed choices about the foods we consume.

Additionally, understanding how to navigate nutrition labels can help us develop a more intuitive relationship with food. Rather than relying solely on external cues such as calorie counts or fat grams, we can tune into our body's internal signals of hunger, fullness, and satisfaction. By eating mindfully and paying attention to how different foods make us feel, we can cultivate a deeper understanding of our nutritional needs and preferences.

Crafting Balanced Meals

Crafting balanced meals is like orchestrating a symphony of flavors, textures, and nutrients—a harmonious blend of ingredients that nourishes both body and soul. It's about creating meals that not only taste delicious but also provide the essential nutrients our bodies need to thrive.

At the heart of crafting balanced meals lies the principle of variety. A balanced meal should include a diverse array of foods from all the major food groups, including fruits, vegetables, whole grains, lean proteins, and healthy fats. Each food group brings its own unique set of nutrients to the table, and by incorporating a variety of foods into our meals, we can ensure that we're getting a broad spectrum of vitamins, minerals, and other essential nutrients.

One key component of balanced meals is incorporating plenty of fruits and vegetables. These nutrient-dense foods are packed with vitamins, minerals, and antioxidants that support overall health and well-being. Aim to fill half of your plate with colorful fruits and vegetables at each meal, choosing a variety of options to maximize nutritional diversity.

In addition to fruits and vegetables, balanced meals should also include a source of lean protein. Protein is essential for building and repairing tissues, supporting immune function, and maintaining muscle mass. Opt for lean protein sources such as poultry, fish, tofu, beans, lentils, and low-fat dairy products, and aim to include a serving of protein with each meal.

Likewise, balanced meals should include whole grains, which provide a rich source of fiber, vitamins, and minerals. Whole grains such as brown rice, quinoa, oats, and whole wheat pasta are less processed and more nutrient-dense than their refined counterparts, making them a healthier choice for supporting overall health and well-being.

Healthy fats are another important component of balanced meals, providing essential fatty acids that support brain health, hormone production, and cell function. Incorporate sources of healthy fats such as avocados, nuts, seeds, olive oil, and fatty fish like salmon and trout into your meals to add flavor and satiety.

Also, it's important to pay attention to portion sizes when crafting balanced meals. While all foods can fit into a balanced diet, it's essential to be mindful of portion sizes to ensure that we're not overeating or under-eating certain foods. Using techniques such as measuring cups, portion control plates, or simply paying attention to hunger and fullness cues can help us achieve the right balance of nutrients without overdoing it.

Crafting balanced meals is an art form that invites us to explore the endless possibilities of flavor, texture, and nutritional composition. It's a creative endeavor that allows us to express our culinary prowess while also nourishing our bodies with the essential nutrients they need to thrive.

One aspect of crafting balanced meals that often goes overlooked is the importance of mindful eating. In today's fast-paced world, it's easy to rush through meals without giving much thought to what or how we're eating. However, taking the time to savor and appreciate each bite can enhance our enjoyment of food and help us tune into our body's hunger and fullness cues. By practicing mindful eating, we can cultivate a deeper connection to our food and foster a greater sense of satisfaction and contentment with our meals.

Furthermore, crafting balanced meals is an opportunity to explore new flavors, ingredients, and culinary techniques. Whether it's experimenting with exotic spices, trying out unfamiliar vegetables, or mastering a new cooking method, there's always something new to discover in the kitchen. By embracing creativity and curiosity, we can keep our meals fresh, exciting, and delicious.

In addition to being delicious, balanced meals should also be practical and convenient. In today's busy world, time is often a scarce commodity, and convenience is key when it comes to meal preparation. Batch cooking, meal prepping, and utilizing time-saving kitchen gadgets can help streamline the cooking process and make it easier to whip up nutritious meals, even on the busiest of days.

Moreover, crafting balanced meals is an opportunity to support local farmers, artisans, and food producers. By sourcing ingredients from local farmers' markets, co-ops, or community-supported agriculture (CSA) programs, we can not only access fresh, seasonal produce but also reduce our carbon footprint and support the local economy. Additionally, buying organic, sustainably sourced, and ethically produced ingredients can further enhance the nutritional quality and environmental sustainability of our meals.

In substance, crafting balanced meals is about more than just putting food on the table—it's about embracing creativity, mindfulness, and connection in our culinary endeavors. By approaching mealtime with intention, joy, and a spirit of adventure, we can transform the act of eating into a deeply enriching and fulfilling experience that nourishes us on multiple levels

CHAPTER 4:Empowering Exercise Regimens

Finding Your Fitness Passion

Finding your fitness passion like discovering a hidden treasure—a journey of exploration, experimentation, and self-discovery that leads to a deeper connection with your body, mind, and spirit. It's about uncovering the activities, movements, and environments that ignite your enthusiasm, invigorate your senses, and bring you joy and fulfillment.

One of the first steps in finding your fitness passion is to explore a variety of activities and modalities. From yoga and Pilates to strength training, running, cycling, dance, martial arts, and beyond, there's a vast array of options to choose from. By sampling different activities and paying attention to how each one makes you feel, you can begin to identify the activities that resonate most deeply with you.

Again, finding your fitness passion involves listening to your body and tuning into its signals and cues. Pay attention to how different activities impact your energy levels, mood, and overall well-being. Notice the activities that leave you feeling energized, inspired, and alive, and prioritize those in your fitness routine.

In addition to exploring different activities, consider experimenting with different environments and settings. Whether it's working out in a gym, exercising outdoors in nature, or joining a group fitness class, the environment can have a significant impact on your enjoyment and engagement with exercise. By finding environments that inspire and motivate you, you can enhance your overall fitness experience.

Furthermore, finding your fitness passion is about embracing variety and spontaneity in your workouts. Instead of sticking to a rigid routine, allow yourself the freedom to mix things up and try new things. Incorporate elements of play, adventure, and exploration into your workouts, and don't be afraid to step outside of your comfort zone.

Another aspect of finding your fitness passion is identifying the deeper motivations and goals that drive your desire to exercise. Ask yourself why you want to be active and what you hope to achieve through your fitness pursuits. Whether it's improving your health, boosting your mood, building strength and endurance, or connecting with others, understanding your underlying motivations can help guide your choices and keep you focused and committed.

Moreover, finding your fitness passion involves embracing the journey of self-discovery and growth that comes with pursuing physical activity. It's about challenging yourself, pushing your limits, and celebrating your successes along the way. Recognize that progress is not always linear and that setbacks and obstacles are a natural part of the process. By approaching your fitness journey with curiosity, resilience, and an open mind, you can continue to evolve and grow as an individual.

Finding your fitness passion is a journey of self-discovery that goes beyond simply finding an activity to do—it's about finding an outlet for self-expression, personal growth, and fulfillment. In today's world, where there are countless fitness trends, programs, and modalities to choose from, discovering what truly resonates with you can feel like searching for a needle in a haystack. However, with patience, curiosity, and an open mind, you can uncover the activities that ignite your passion and bring you a sense of joy and purpose.

One approach to finding your fitness passion is to draw inspiration from your interests, hobbies, and personality traits. Consider activities that align with your values, preferences, and natural inclinations. For example, if you enjoy spending time outdoors, you might explore hiking, trail running, or outdoor yoga. If you thrive in social settings, group fitness classes or team sports might be a better fit for you. By tapping into what you already love and enjoy, you can increase the likelihood of finding a fitness activity that resonates with you on a deeper level.

Again, finding your fitness passion involves being open to trying new things and stepping outside of your comfort zone. While it's natural to gravitate towards familiar activities, it's important to challenge yourself to explore new possibilities and experiences. Consider taking a class or workshop in a discipline you've never tried before, or joining a community or club centered around a particular activity. By exposing yourself to new ideas and perspectives, you expand your horizons and increase your chances of discovering something that truly captivates you.

In addition to exploring different activities, consider the role that movement plays in your life outside of formal exercise. Pay attention to the activities that bring you joy, whether it's dancing around the house, playing with your kids or pets, or exploring new places on foot or by bike. These everyday movements can offer valuable insights into the types of activities that resonate with you on a deeper level and can serve as inspiration for finding your fitness passion.

Furthermore, finding your fitness passion involves being attuned to your body and its signals. Notice how different activities make you feel physically, mentally, and emotionally. Pay attention to the activities that leave you feeling energized, inspired, and fulfilled, and seek out opportunities to incorporate more of those activities into your routine. Conversely, be mindful of activities that feel draining, stressful, or unfulfilling, and consider whether they align with your true passions and interests.

Another aspect of finding your fitness passion is recognizing that it's okay to change and evolve over time. Your interests, preferences, and goals may shift as you grow and develop as an individual, and that's perfectly normal. Be open to exploring new avenues and revisiting old passions, and allow yourself the freedom to adapt and pivot as needed. By embracing change and remaining open to new possibilities, you create space for continued growth and discovery in your fitness journey.

Incorporating Movement into Daily Life

Incorporating movement into daily life is about embracing the concept of "movement as medicine"—recognizing that physical activity is not just something we do at the gym or during structured workouts, but an essential component of overall health and well-being that can and should be integrated into every aspect of our daily routines. It's about finding creative ways to stay active throughout the day, regardless of our schedule, commitments, or environment.

One of the simplest ways to incorporate movement into daily life is to make small, intentional changes to your daily habits and routines. For example, take the stairs instead of the elevator, park farther away from your destination to get in some extra steps, or stand up and stretch periodically throughout the day if you have a desk job. These small changes may seem insignificant on their own, but over time, they can add up to significant improvements in your overall activity level and health.

Finding opportunities to move throughout the day doesn't have to be limited to traditional forms of exercise. Everyday activities such as walking the dog, gardening, playing with your kids or grandkids, or cleaning the house can all provide valuable opportunities to get your body moving and increase your daily activity levels. By reframing these activities as opportunities for movement and physical activity, you can turn everyday tasks into opportunities for improving your health and well-being.

In addition to incorporating movement into your daily routines, consider finding activities that you genuinely enjoy and look forward to doing. Whether it's dancing, cycling, hiking, practicing yoga, or playing a sport, finding activities that bring you joy and fulfillment can make it easier to stay motivated and committed to regular physical activity. Experiment with different activities to find what resonates with you, and don't be afraid to try new things or step outside of your comfort zone.

Furthermore, incorporating movement into daily life is about being creative and resourceful with your time and environment. Look for opportunities to multitask and combine physical activity with other tasks or activities you need to do. For example, listen to an audiobook or podcast while going for a walk or run, or use a standing desk or stability ball at work to keep your body engaged and active throughout the day.

Another effective strategy for incorporating movement into daily life is to prioritize activities that align with your interests, goals, and values. If you're passionate about environmental conservation, for example, you might choose to participate in activities like hiking, biking, or volunteering for outdoor clean-up efforts. By integrating activities that align with your passions and values, you can infuse your movement practice with a sense of purpose and meaning that goes beyond just physical exercise.

Also, incorporating movement into daily life is not just about physical health—it's also about nurturing your mental, emotional, and spiritual well-being. Movement has been shown to have numerous benefits for mental health, including reducing stress, anxiety, and depression, improving mood and self-esteem, and enhancing cognitive function and creativity. By prioritizing activities that nourish your mind and spirit as well as your body, you can create a holistic approach to health and well-being that supports your overall quality of life.

Incorporating movement into daily life is a holistic approach to wellness that extends beyond just physical health. It's about recognizing the interconnectedness of our bodies, minds, and spirits and embracing movement as a tool for promoting overall well-being and vitality.

One way to incorporate movement into daily life is by fostering a mindset of mindfulness and intentionality. Instead of viewing physical activity as something separate from the rest of our lives, we can approach each moment as an opportunity to move and engage our bodies.

Whether it's taking a mindful walk in nature, practicing yoga or tai chi, or simply paying attention to our posture and alignment as we go about our daily tasks, mindfulness can help us stay present and connected to our bodies throughout the day.

Again, incorporating movement into daily life is about finding balance and flexibility in our approach to physical activity. While structured workouts and exercise routines certainly have their place, it's important to recognize that movement doesn't have to be rigid or regimented. By allowing ourselves the freedom to move in ways that feel good and nourishing, we can cultivate a more intuitive and sustainable approach to fitness that honors our body's needs and preferences.

Another key aspect of incorporating movement into daily life is creating an environment that supports an active lifestyle. This might involve making small changes to our surroundings, such as rearranging furniture to create more space for movement, investing in ergonomic equipment or tools that promote good posture and alignment, or setting aside designated areas for physical activity and exercise. By creating a supportive environment that encourages movement and activity, we can make it easier to incorporate physical activity into our daily routines.

Furthermore, incorporating movement into daily life is about fostering a sense of joy and playfulness in our approach to physical activity. Instead of viewing exercise as a chore or obligation, we can approach it with a spirit of curiosity, exploration, and creativity. Whether it's trying out a new dance class, playing a game of frisbee with friends, or simply taking a moment to skip or jump for joy, finding ways to infuse movement with fun and spontaneity can make it more enjoyable and sustainable in the long run.

Moreover, incorporating movement into daily life is about recognizing that every little bit counts. While it's easy to get caught up in the idea that we need to engage in long, intense workouts to reap the benefits of physical activity, the truth is that even small amounts of movement can have a significant impact on our health and well-being. Whether it's taking the scenic route on your daily commute, doing a few stretches while waiting for the kettle to boil, or dancing around the kitchen while cooking dinner, finding creative ways to sneak in extra movement throughout the day can add up to big benefits over time.

In substance, incorporating movement into daily life is about adopting a holistic approach to health and well-being that recognizes the importance of physical activity in all aspects of our lives. By fostering mindfulness, balance, joy, and creativity in our approach to movement, we can create a lifestyle that supports our overall health, happiness, and vitality. Whether it's finding moments of stillness and presence in our daily activities or infusing our movement practice with playfulness and spontaneity, every step we take towards incorporating movement into our daily lives brings us one step closer to living our most vibrant and fulfilling life.

CHAPTER 5:Mindset Mastery

Cultivating Self-Compassion

Cultivating self-compassion is a journey of self-discovery, acceptance, and kindness—a journey that invites us to embrace our humanity with gentleness and understanding. It's about recognizing our inherent worth and value as human beings, regardless of our flaws, imperfections, or mistakes. By nurturing a compassionate relationship with ourselves, we can cultivate greater resilience, inner peace, and well-being in our lives.

One of the foundational elements of cultivating self-compassion is developing a sense of mindfulness—being present and aware of our thoughts, feelings, and experiences without judgment or criticism. Mindfulness allows us to observe our inner landscape with curiosity and compassion, recognizing that all human beings experience pain, suffering, and challenges as part of the human condition. By cultivating mindfulness, we can create space for self-compassion to flourish and grow.

Again, cultivating self-compassion involves adopting a mindset of kindness and understanding towards ourselves. Instead of berating ourselves for our perceived shortcomings or failures, we can offer ourselves the same warmth, care, and support that we would offer to a dear friend or loved one. This might involve speaking to ourselves with words of encouragement and affirmation, practicing self-care and self-soothing activities, or simply offering ourselves a gentle touch or hug in moments of distress.

In addition to kindness, cultivating self-compassion requires us to embrace the concept of common humanity—the understanding that we are not alone in our struggles and that all human beings experience pain, suffering, and vulnerability at various points in their lives. By recognizing our shared humanity, we can cultivate greater empathy and compassion towards ourselves and others, fostering a sense of connection and belonging that is essential for well-being.

Furthermore, cultivating self-compassion involves letting go of the myth of perfectionism—the belief that we must be flawless, faultless, and infallible in order to be worthy of love and acceptance. Instead, we can embrace our humanity with all its messy, imperfect beauty, recognizing that our worthiness is not contingent on our achievements, successes, or external validation. By letting go of perfectionism and embracing our inherent worthiness, we can create space for self-compassion to flourish and thrive.

Another important aspect of cultivating self-compassion is practicing self-forgiveness—the act of letting go of resentment, bitterness, and self-blame and embracing forgiveness, understanding, and grace towards ourselves. This can be a challenging process, especially if we carry deep wounds or traumas from our past, but it is essential for healing and growth. By releasing ourselves from the burden of self-condemnation and embracing self-forgiveness, we can cultivate greater peace, freedom, and well-being in our lives.

Moreover, cultivating self-compassion involves nurturing a sense of resilience—the ability to bounce back from adversity, setbacks, and challenges with grace and strength. Self-compassion provides a powerful buffer against stress, anxiety, and depression, helping us navigate life's ups and downs with greater ease and resilience. By cultivating self-compassion, we can build a solid foundation of inner strength and resilience that supports us in facing life's challenges with courage, dignity, and grace.

ongoing journey that requires patience, persistence, and practice. It's not something that happens overnight, but rather a gradual process of learning to relate to ourselves with greater kindness, gentleness, and understanding. As we navigate life's challenges and uncertainties, cultivating self-compassion provides us with a powerful anchor—a source of inner strength and resilience that helps us weather the storms and navigate the highs and lows with grace and dignity.

Moreover, cultivating self-compassion is not about avoiding difficult emotions or pretending that everything is fine. It's about embracing our full range of human experiences, including pain, sorrow, fear, and doubt, with an open heart and a compassionate mind. By acknowledging and validating our emotions without judgment or resistance, we create space for healing, growth, and transformation to occur.

Furthermore, cultivating self-compassion involves learning to set healthy boundaries and prioritize our own well-being. This means saying no to activities, relationships, and obligations that drain our energy or compromise our values, and saying yes to self-care, self-expression, and self-fulfillment. By honoring our own needs and desires, we cultivate a deep sense of self-respect and self-worth that forms the foundation of self-compassion.

In addition, cultivating self-compassion involves letting go of comparison and competition and embracing our own unique journey and path. It's about recognizing that we are all on our own individual paths, with our own strengths, weaknesses, and challenges, and that there is no one-size-fits-all approach to success or happiness. By celebrating our differences and honoring our unique gifts and talents, we create a more inclusive and compassionate world where everyone can thrive.

Moreover, cultivating self-compassion requires us to practice self-care and self-nurturing on a regular basis. This might involve engaging in activities that bring us joy and fulfillment, such as spending time in nature, pursuing creative hobbies, or connecting with loved ones. It might also involve setting aside time for rest, relaxation, and rejuvenation, allowing ourselves to recharge and replenish our energy reserves.

Cultivating self-compassion is an ongoing journey that requires patience, persistence, and practice. It's not something that happens overnight, but rather a gradual process of learning to relate to ourselves with greater kindness, gentleness, and understanding. As we navigate life's challenges and uncertainties, cultivating self-compassion provides us with a powerful anchor—a source of inner strength and resilience that helps us weather the storms and navigate the highs and lows with grace and dignity.

Again, cultivating self-compassion is not about avoiding difficult emotions or pretending that everything is fine. It's about embracing our full range of human experiences, including pain, sorrow, fear, and doubt, with an open heart and a compassionate mind. By acknowledging and validating our emotions without judgment or resistance, we create space for healing, growth, and transformation to occur.

Furthermore, cultivating self-compassion involves learning to set healthy boundaries and prioritize our own well-being. This means saying no to activities, relationships, and obligations that drain our energy or compromise our values, and saying yes to self-care, self-expression, and self-fulfillment. By honoring our own needs and desires, we cultivate a deep sense of self-respect and self-worth that forms the foundation of self-compassion.

In addition, cultivating self-compassion involves letting go of comparison and competition and embracing our own unique journey and path. It's about recognizing that we are all on our own individual paths, with our own strengths, weaknesses, and challenges, and that there is no one-size-fits-all approach to success or happiness. By celebrating our differences and honoring our unique gifts and talents, we create a more inclusive and compassionate world where everyone can thrive. Moreover, cultivating self-compassion requires us to practice self-care and self-nurturing on a regular basis. This might involve engaging in activities that bring us joy and fulfillment, such as spending time in nature, pursuing creative hobbies, or connecting with loved ones. It might also involve setting aside time for rest, relaxation, and rejuvenation, allowing ourselves to recharge and replenish our energy reserves.

Overcoming Plateaus and Setbacks

Overcoming plateaus and setbacks is an essential part of any journey towards personal growth, achievement, and success. Whether we're striving to improve our fitness, advance in our careers, or pursue our passions and dreams, we're likely to encounter obstacles, challenges, and setbacks along the way. While these setbacks can be discouraging and frustrating, they also present valuable opportunities for learning, growth, and resilience-building.

One of the first steps in overcoming plateaus and setbacks is to adopt a mindset of resilience and perseverance. Instead of viewing setbacks as failures or reasons to give up, see them as temporary roadblocks on the path to success. Embrace the idea that setbacks are a natural and inevitable part of any journey towards growth and achievement, and that they provide valuable opportunities for learning, adaptation, and growth.

Moreover, overcoming plateaus and setbacks involves reframing our perspective and focusing on the lessons and insights that can be gained from our experiences. Instead of dwelling on what went wrong or assigning blame, ask yourself what you can learn from the experience and how you can use that knowledge to improve and grow moving forward. By approaching setbacks with curiosity, openness, and a willingness to learn, you can transform them into stepping stones towards future success.

Again, overcoming plateaus and setbacks requires us to practice self-compassion and self-acceptance. It's natural to feel disappointed, frustrated, or discouraged when things don't go as planned, but beating ourselves up or dwelling on our shortcomings only serves to undermine our confidence and motivation. Instead, offer yourself the same kindness, understanding, and support that you would offer to a friend or loved one facing similar challenges. Treat yourself with compassion and gentleness, and remember that setbacks are a normal and unavoidable part of the human experience.

Furthermore, overcoming plateaus and setbacks often involves seeking support and guidance from others. Whether it's reaching out to a mentor, coach, or trusted friend for advice and encouragement, or seeking out resources and tools to help you navigate challenges more effectively, don't be afraid to ask for help when you need it. Surround yourself with people who believe in you and your abilities, and lean on their support and guidance as you work through setbacks and obstacles.

Likewise, overcoming plateaus and setbacks requires us to be flexible and adaptable in our approach to problem-solving and goal-setting. If a particular strategy or approach isn't yielding the desired results, be willing to reassess, adjust, and try something new. Experiment with different techniques, methods, and approaches until you find what works best for you, and be open to feedback and input from others along the way.

Overcoming plateaus and setbacks is a deeply personal journey that challenges us to dig deep, confront our fears, and tap into our inner reserves of strength and resilience. It's a journey that requires us to confront our limitations, confront our fears, and confront our doubts head-on, and to emerge stronger, wiser, and more resilient on the other side.

One of the keys to overcoming plateaus and setbacks is to cultivate a growth mindset—a belief that our abilities and intelligence are not fixed, but can be developed through effort, perseverance, and learning. By adopting a growth mindset, we can approach challenges with a sense of curiosity and optimism, viewing setbacks as opportunities for growth and learning rather than insurmountable obstacles. This mindset shift empowers us to embrace challenges knowing that each setback brings us onewith courage and resilience, step closer to our goals.

Also, overcoming plateaus and setbacks involves developing a strong sense of self-awareness and emotional intelligence. It's important to recognize when we're feeling stuck or discouraged and to acknowledge and honor our emotions without judgment or criticism. By cultivating self-awareness and emotional intelligence, we can better understand the underlying causes of our setbacks and develop effective strategies for overcoming them. This might involve practicing mindfulness, journaling, or seeking support from a therapist or coach to help us navigate difficult emotions and experiences.

In addition, overcoming plateaus and setbacks requires us to cultivate a sense of perseverance and determination in the face of adversity. It's easy to become discouraged or disheartened when things don't go as planned, but it's essential to stay focused on our long-term goals and to keep moving forward, one step at a time. By maintaining a sense of determination and perseverance, we can overcome even the most daunting challenges and emerge stronger and more resilient on the other side.

Furthermore, overcoming plateaus and setbacks often involves embracing the concept of radical self-acceptance—the idea that we are worthy and deserving of love and acceptance exactly as we are, flaws and all. Instead of striving for perfection or comparing ourselves to others, we can embrace our humanity with compassion and kindness, recognizing that our worthiness is not contingent on our achievements or successes. By practicing radical self-acceptance, we can cultivate a deep sense of inner peace and contentment that empowers us to navigate setbacks with grace and resilience.

In essence, overcoming plateaus and setbacks requires us to cultivate a sense of gratitude and appreciation for the lessons and blessings that come from adversity. While setbacks can be painful and challenging, they also provide valuable opportunities for growth, learning, and self-discovery.

By embracing setbacks as opportunities for growth and transformation, we can cultivate a sense of gratitude and appreciation for the richness and complexity of the human experience.

CHAPTER 6: Strategies for Sustainable Success

Meal Prepping and Planning

Meal prepping and planning is a powerful tool for optimizing nutrition, saving time, and reducing stress in our busy lives. It involves preparing meals and snacks in advance, usually at the beginning of the week, and portioning them out into containers for easy storage and access throughout the week. By taking the time to plan and prepare our meals ahead of time, we can ensure that we have nutritious, delicious options readily available, even on our busiest days.One of the key benefits of meal prepping and planning is that it allows us to take control of our nutrition and make healthier choices. When we have healthy meals and snacks prepped and ready to go, we're less likely to reach for convenience foods or unhealthy options when hunger strikes. Instead, we can reach for a nutritious, balanced meal that supports our health and well-being, helping us stay energized and focused throughout the day.

Moreover, meal prepping and planning can help us save time and money in the long run. By preparing meals in bulk and portioning them out ahead of time, we can streamline our cooking process and reduce the amount of time spent in the kitchen each day. This can be especially helpful for busy individuals and families who may not have the time or energy to cook elaborate meals from scratch every day. Additionally, by buying ingredients in bulk and planning meals in advance, we can save money on groceries and reduce food waste, as we're less likely to buy ingredients that we don't end up using.

In addition to saving time and money, meal prepping and planning can also help reduce stress and simplify our lives. When we know exactly what we're going to eat for each meal and snack throughout the week, we can eliminate the need to make last-minute decisions about what to eat, which can be a significant source of stress for many people. Additionally, having meals prepped and ready to go can reduce the mental load associated with meal planning and preparation, freeing up mental energy for other tasks and activities.

Likewise, meal prepping and planning can help us stay on track with our health and fitness goals. By preparing meals that are aligned with our nutritional needs and goals, we can ensure that we're fueling our bodies with the nutrients they need to perform at their best. Whether we're trying to lose weight, build muscle, or improve our overall health, meal prepping and planning can provide us with the structure and consistency we need to stay on track and make progress towards our goals.

Another benefit of meal prepping and planning is that it can help us develop healthier eating habits over time. When we have nutritious meals and snacks readily available, we're more likely to make healthy choices throughout the day, even when we're busy or stressed. Additionally, by experimenting with new recipes and ingredients during the meal prepping process, we can expand our culinary repertoire and discover new foods and flavors that we enjoy, making healthy eating more enjoyable and sustainable in the long run.

Besides, meal prepping and planning can be a great way to involve the whole family in meal preparation and cooking. By getting everyone involved in the process of planning and preparing meals, we can foster a sense of teamwork and cooperation, and teach valuable life skills to children and teenagers. Additionally, involving family members in meal prepping and planning can help ensure that everyone's preferences and dietary needs are taken into account, making mealtime more enjoyable and inclusive for everyone.

Meal prepping and planning is a lifestyle choice that goes beyond just saving time and money—it's about taking ownership of our health and well-being and making intentional choices that support our goals and priorities. By investing time and effort into meal prepping and planning, we're making a commitment to ourselves and our health, and setting ourselves up for success in all areas of our lives.

Moreover, meal prepping and planning can be a powerful tool for building self-discipline and consistency. By establishing a routine of planning and preparing meals ahead of time, we're creating structure and accountability in our lives, which can help us stay focused and disciplined in pursuit of our goals. Whether we're trying to eat healthier, lose weight, or improve our fitness, meal prepping and planning can provide us with the framework and support we need to stay on track and make progress towards our goals.

Additionally, meal prepping and planning can help us develop a healthier relationship with food and eating. When we take the time to plan and prepare meals that are aligned with our nutritional needs and goals, we're sending a powerful message to ourselves that we value our health and well-being. This can help shift our mindset around food from one of deprivation and restriction to one of abundance and nourishment, empowering us to make choices that support our health and vitality.

Also, meal prepping and planning can be a form of self-care and self-love. By taking the time to plan and prepare meals that nourish our bodies and support our goals, we're demonstrating a commitment to ourselves and our well-being. This act of self-care can have ripple effects throughout our lives, helping us feel more energized, focused, and empowered to tackle whatever challenges come our way.

In addition, meal prepping and planning can be a source of creativity and inspiration in the kitchen. By experimenting with new recipes, flavors, and ingredients during the meal prepping process, we can expand our culinary horizons and discover new foods and flavors that we enjoy. This can make healthy eating more enjoyable and sustainable in the long run, as we're constantly discovering new ways to nourish and delight our taste buds.

Moreover, meal prepping and planning can be a form of mindfulness practice, helping us stay present and engaged in the moment as we plan and prepare meals with intention and purpose. By focusing our attention on the task at hand and savoring the process of creating nourishing meals for ourselves and our loved ones, we can cultivate a deeper sense of gratitude, contentment, and fulfillment in our lives.

Staying Motivated for the Long Haul

Staying motivated for the long haul is a journey that, and a deep sense of purpose. Whether we're pursuing personal or professional goals, embarking on a new fitness regimen, or striving to make positive changes in our lives, maintaining motivation over the long term can be challenging. However, by cultivating certain habits, mindset shifts, and strategies, we can fuel our motivation and sustain our momentum even in the face of obstacles and setbacks.

The key to staying motivated for the long haul is to cultivate a clear sense of purpose and direction. When we have a compelling reason why we're pursuing our goals, we're more likely to stay committed and resilient in the face of challenges. Take the time to reflect on your values, passions, and aspirations, and identify the deeper purpose behind your goals. Whether it's improving your health, making a positive impact in the world, or pursuing your dreams, clarifying your purpose can provide you with a powerful source of motivation and inspiration to keep going, even when the going gets tough.

Moreover, staying motivated for the long haul involves setting realistic, achievable goals that are aligned with your values and priorities. Break down your long-term goals into smaller, manageable milestones, and celebrate your progress along the way. By setting realistic goals and acknowledging your achievements, you can build momentum and confidence over time, fueling your motivation to keep moving forward.

Likewise,to setting goals, staying motivated for the long haul requires us to cultivate a growth mindset—a belief that our abilities and intelligence are not fixed, but can be developed through effort, perseverance, and learning. Embrace challenges as opportunities for growth and learning, and view setbacks as temporary obstacles on the path to success. By adopting a growth mindset, you can stay resilient and motivated in the face of adversity, and continue to progress towards your goals with determination and resilience.

Also, staying motivated for the long haul involves creating a supportive environment that fosters your growth and development. Surround yourself with positive, encouraging people who believe in you and your abilities, and seek out mentors, coaches, or role models who can provide guidance and support along the way. Additionally, eliminate distractions and obstacles that may undermine your motivation, and create systems and routines that support your progress and success.

As well, staying motivated for the long haul requires us to take care of our physical, mental, and emotional well-being. Prioritize self-care activities that replenish your energy and nourish your soul, such as exercise, meditation, journaling, or spending time in nature. Practice self-compassion and kindness towards yourself, and be gentle with yourself during times of difficulty or struggle. By prioritizing your well-being and honoring your needs, you can sustain your motivation and resilience over the long term.

In addition, staying motivated for the long haul involves staying connected to your goals and vision, even when the going gets tough. Visualize your success, and remind yourself of the reasons why you embarked on this journey in the first place. Surround yourself with reminders of your goals and aspirations, whether it's a vision board, a written manifesto, or a simple mantra that inspires you. By staying connected to your goals and vision, you can stay motivated and focused on the path ahead, even when faced with challenges and setbacks.

Staying motivated for the long haul involves cultivating a mindset of resilience and adaptability. Life is full of unexpected twists and turns, and staying motivated for the long term requires us to be flexible and open to change. Instead of viewing setbacks or obstacles as roadblocks, see them as opportunities for growth and learning. Embrace challenges as opportunities to develop new skills, gain new perspectives, and become stronger and more resilient versions of ourselves.

Again, staying motivated for the long haul involves finding balance in our lives. It's important to prioritize our goals and aspirations, but it's also essential to make time for rest, relaxation, and rejuvenation. Burnout and exhaustion can quickly drain our motivation and energy, so it's crucial to listen to our bodies and minds and give ourselves the care and nourishment we need to thrive. Make self-care a priority, and create space in your life for activities that bring you joy, fulfillment, and peace of mind.

Also, staying motivated for the long haul involves staying connected to our passions and interests. When we're passionate about something, we're naturally more motivated to pursue it with vigor and enthusiasm. Take time to explore your interests, try new things, and pursue activities that bring you joy and fulfillment. Whether it's a hobby, a creative project, or a cause you're passionate about, staying connected to your passions can fuel your motivation and keep you inspired for the long journey ahead.

Again ,staying motivated for the long haul involves seeking support and guidance from others. We don't have to navigate our journey alone—there are countless resources and communities available to support us along the way. Whether it's joining a support group, working with a mentor or coach, or simply reaching out to friends and loved ones for encouragement and advice, don't hesitate to lean on others for support when you need it. Surround yourself with positive, uplifting people who believe in you and your abilities, and let their support fuel your motivation and determination.

CONCLUSION

In embracing your new life, you 're not just embarking on a trip of physical metamorphosis, but a profound shift towards holistic well- being and tone- discovery. Throughout' Time to Trim Down', we have uncovered the tools, strategies, and perceptivity demanded to embark on this transformative trip with confidence and determination. By recognizing patterns and triggers, prostrating emotional eating, and demystifying metabolism, you've gained inestimable knowledge about your body and mind. You've learned to establish realistic pretensions, navigate nutrition markers, and craft balanced refections that nourish and energize you from the inside out. But beyond the figures on the scale or the size of your jeans, embracing your new life is about embracing a mindset of tone- compassion, adaptability, and growth. It's about recognizing that heartiness isn't a destination, but a trip — one that requires tolerance, perseverance, and a amenability to embrace change. As you continue on this trip, remember to celebrate your progress, no matter how small. Each healthy choice you make, each handicap you overcome, is a testament to your strength and commitment to yourself. Embrace the ups and campo, the triumphs and lapses, knowing that each step forward brings you near to the vibrant, fulfilling life you deserve. In the end,' Time to Trim Down' isn't just about losing weight — it's about gaining a newfound sense of confidence, vitality, and tone- love. It's about reclaiming your health and happiness, and embracing the measureless eventuality within you. So as you step into your new life, remember to embrace it with open arms, knowing that the stylish is yet to come. Then is to your trip of metamorphosis, commission, and tone- discovery — may it be filled with endless possibilities and bottomless joy.